A COUNTRY DOCTOR

SMALL TOWN MEDICAL PRACTICE
IN THE NINETEEN SIXTIES

DON L. ERVIN, MD

ISBN: 1470009641
ISBN 13: 9781470009649

In memory of my parents,
Mark K. and Pearl Sylvia Ervin,
who made it possible for me to become a doctor.

INTRODUCTION

Even as a child, I knew that I wanted to be a doctor and assumed that someday I would be. I was probably influenced by my father who greatly admired his grandfather, Dr. James R. Scott. Dr. Scott had been a doctor in the civil war and continued to practice for many years in the very small Illinois town where my father was born.

I was a mediocre student in grade school and was surprised when I made straight A' s during my first term in high school. I continued to make A's and B's through high school and college. For some years after World War II the medical schools were flooded with applications from veterans on the GI Bill, and they only accepted students with A or A+ averages. Fortunately for me, the Illinois Agricultural Association had some kind of deal with the University of Illinois College of Medicine whereby the university would reserve eleven places in each freshman class for students who would agree to practice for at least five years in rural Illinois towns with less than 5,000 population. I was lucky enough to secure one of those places.

I actually did well in medical school and finished in the upper third (just barely) of my class. Most of my junior year was spent at the Cook County Hospital, which was a veritable zoo. It was a huge, dirty institution where one could see almost every malady known to man. I also spent about three months at nearby Presbyterian Hospital on the surgical service. In 1954, Presbyterian failed to fill its quota of interns and made a deal with the university to take six senior students to act as interns, and these students would get credit for their fourth year of medical school. I was selected as one of those six students. In effect, I had a year of internship before I finished medical school, but I still needed an official internship to qualify for a license to practice.

During the years that followed, I had many interesting experiences. This writing is to recount some of the more unusual ones. Some of these stories may be hard to believe, but I know that every word I have written is true, except that I have altered some names "to protect the innocent".

Another reason for writing is to point out the extreme changes we have seen in medical care and its cost over the past fifty years.

INTERNSHIP

After four years of living on Chicago's Near West Side while attending medical school, I was anxious to get away from the crowded, noisy city, as was my new wife, who had been raised in a small town about 30 miles west of Chicago. Accordingly, I applied for an internship at St. Joseph's Hospital in Marshfield, Wisconsin and was accepted. Marshfield was, at that time, a city of about 30,000 in central Wisconsin. The internship was sponsored by the Marshfield Clinic, a group, then, of thirty two respected physicians in various specialties. Since there were no residents at St Joseph's the interns, six of us, were given a lot of responsibility. I needed that because I intended to do general practice in a small town in southern Illinois. It was a very hard year.

St. Joseph's was a 250 bed catholic hospital operated by a community of nuns called the Sisters of The Sorrowful Mother. The sisters' habits completely covered their bodies except for their faces and hands. Like most good-sized hospitals there was a school of nursing. I don't think any of the students were nuns. Most of the sisters were easy to get along with, and the atmosphere was pretty congenial. Each of the interns spent every day, every third night and every third weekend at the hospital, except the one on the OB service who stayed at the hospital all week but was off weekends. We probably needed at least ten interns, so the six of us worked very hard. We were paid $250 per month.

The medical staff mostly comprised the Marshfield Clinic doctors, but also included several general practitioners from surrounding small towns. The interns were, for the most part, treated reasonably well.

GOOSE - NECK LAMP DEFIBRILLATOR

On my third day as an intern I was watching Dr. Ben Lawton do a bronchoscopy. In those days that involved shoving a rigid tube down the patient's throat into the trachea and, hopefully, into one and then the other main bronchus. Flexible fiberoptic medical instruments didn't become available until about twelve years later. It was a pretty brutal procedure.

As Dr. Lawton was withdrawing the bronchoscope the patient went into cardiac arrest. I should explain here that closed chest cardiac resuscitation wasn't recognized until the early sixties. In 1955 the only treatment for cardiac arrest was to cut open the chest, grasp the heart between both hands and rhythmically squeeze it, which is exactly what Dr. Lawton did. He told me to pick up the knife and cut the costal cartilages at the upper end of his incision so he could get a better grip on the heart. After I did that he opened the pericardium and saw that the heart was fibrillating, i.e. wriggling all over instead of contracting effectively. The only effective treatment for ventricular fibrillation is to apply an electric shock to the heart, which is usually followed by a resumption of a regular rhythm. This is usually done with a sophisticated instrument, a defibrillator, which controls the amount and duration of the shock. In 1955 there was no defibrillator within one hundred miles of Marshfield.

By this time the hospital's only anesthesiologist had arrived and was bagging the patient, i.e. breathing for him with an anesthesia machine. The three of us discussed possible courses of action and decided that there was only one. Dr. Lawton told me to pick up the knife again and cut the long cord off a nearby goose-neck lamp then strip the insulation off about one inch of the cut end and separate the wires for about ten inches, which I did. He was all the while massaging the heart. I handed the wire to him, and he held the two bare ends against the heart and told me to plug the wire in and out of a nearby wall socket "real quick". I did that, and the heart resumed normal beating. I guess Dr. Lawton was careful to keep his fingers away from the bare ends of the wires since he wasn't electrocuted. I wish I could say that the patient recovered, but he didn't. He had just gone too long without adequate circulation.

A BOARD IN THE HEAD

One afternoon when I was coming out of the emergency room I saw three men walking toward me. The one in the middle was a short, stocky, bowlegged man in his mid fifties with a foot long board sticking out of his head. The board was about 1 inch wide and ¾ of an inch thick. I was told that he worked in a lumber yard and that the board had flown out of a machine and hit him in the head. We put him on a table, and I thought about what to do next. I concluded that people shouldn't have boards sticking out of their heads and decided to give it one good pull to see if it would come out. I did, and it didn't, so I decided to call for help, (which I should have done in the first place).

After Dr. Lawton arrived we prepped and anesthetized the man in the operating room and made short incisions on each side of where the board had penetrated the scalp. We saw that it had not penetrated the skull but had "splattered" into splinters between the scalp and the skull which is why I couldn't pull it out. We dissected the splinters free from the tissue overlying the skull and cleaned and closed the wound. The man made a complete, uneventful recovery. In my mind I can still see that little bowlegged man walking down the hall with a board sticking out of his head.

MY FIRST TRACHEOTOMY

Dr. Charlie Veddar didn't have much formal surgical training beyond internship, but he probably did a lot of combat surgery during world war two while attached to the Tenth Mountain Division in Italy. Up until the late sixties it was still possible to become a "self-made surgeon" by learning from older colleagues and through study and experience (as I later did). In any case he was one of three general surgeons with the Marshfield Clinic when I arrived there. He was very competent and meticulous and his work was almost artistic.

I assisted him one morning when he did a subtotal thyroidectomy and, as usual, the surgical site looked almost natural when he finished. Late that afternoon I was called to the patient's room and found her unconscious and struggling for breath. Her neck was swollen, and it was obvious that postoperative bleeding had compressed her trachea. The astute nurses already had a knife and tracheotomy set at the bedside. I promptly cut the sutures, opened the wound, cut a hole in the trachea and inserted a tracheotomy tube. The patient resumed normal breathing and regained consciousness. Soon after that Dr. Veddar arrived and did his best to restore his pristine surgery which I had messed up. He later grudgingly agreed that the patient would have died had I not done what I did. Most experienced surgeons would find nothing noteworthy about this episode, but I was not an experienced surgeon. I had never even seen anyone do a tracheotomy before, so it was very noteworthy to me.

FINGERNAIL HEART SURGERY

Dr. Ben Lawton was a certified thoracic surgeon, just out of the army before joining the Marshfield Clinic. He was a stocky, unpretentious man and an aggressive surgeon, that is, he would try anything to keep a patient alive, even if it meant cutting off the entire lower half of their body, as it did in one case. What little heart surgery was done in the mid fifties was done by thoracic surgeons, and the most common procedure was a mitral valvulotomy, i.e. attempting to open a stenotic or constricted mitral heart valve which had been damaged by rheumatic fever, which was still common at that time. The mitral valve is located between the left upper and lower chambers of the heart, i.e. the atrium and the ventrical, and a little pouch called the auricle protrudes from the atrium. The accepted procedure at that time was to expose the heart and put a purse string suture around the auricle. The surgeon would then remove the surgical glove from his right hand, cut off the tip of the auricle and stick his index finger into it while the assistant held the purse string tight around his finger. He would then "break" the stenotic valve with his fingernail, withdraw his finger and put on a fresh glove while the assistant closed the auricle with the purse string. Today, in 2011, most people would not believe this, but I have seen it done.

INDEX FINGER IV

Because of my year of externship at Presbyterian Hospital in Chicago, I had a lot of experience in starting IVs, and I was pretty good at it before I started my internship. My crowning achievement in that regard involved a patient who had required so many IVs that he had almost no suitable veins left. I was able to get an IV into a vein in his index finger and ran two liters of fluid through it before it infiltrated. It was a minor thing, but anyone familiar with starting IVs will understand why I am still proud of it.

CATATONIC CONSTIPATION

There was a state mental asylum about ten miles south of Marshfield. In those days such places were very heavily populated since there was no alternative for warehousing people who were severely insane. A newly assigned "in-house" doctor there discovered that one of his patients, a catatonic schizophrenic, had a colostomy for no discernible reason. He sent her to the Marshfield Clinic to see if her colostomy should be "taken down" which would restore normal bowel function. When a barium enema showed no reason for a colostomy Dr. Walt Kearny, the third general surgeon at the clinic, decided that we should do it. Walt had just finished his residency at the Hines VA hospital near Chicago and was a very competent surgeon. The patient was completely unable to communicate and constantly stared intently at something on her left which she could see but we couldn't. After Dr. Kearny took down her colostomy we found out why she had it. For whatever reason, she absolutely would not have a bowel movement despite laxatives and enemas. I can't imagine how she did it, but nothing could make her have a normal BM. After several days we restored her colostomy and sent her back to the asylum.

BLASPHEMOUS HYMN SINGING

One of our elderly patients at Marshfield had suffered a severe stroke which left him aphasic, i.e. unable to talk except for one word, which was goddamn. He could still carry a tune, and his very religious wife spent a lot of time at his bedside singing hymns with him. It was a little strange to hear him singing "goddamn, goddamn" to the tune of Amazing Grace.

RUINED SHOES

In the early spring a big 60 some year old man was brought in perspiring profusely and complaining of abdominal pain. His abdomen was distended and rigid, and he had a history of peptic ulcer. We found X-ray evidence of air under the diaphragm and concluded that his ulcer had perforated several days before his admission. I can't imagine how he endured the pain for two or three days, but he was a tough old German. When we got the patient to surgery Dr. Lawton told the anesthetist to tip the table a few degrees toward me before he made his incision. Knowing his morbid sense of humor I should have suspected something, but I didn't. When he made a long, deep incision about a half gallon of foul pus spewed out all over my gown, pants and shoes. After we had finished the operation and I had discarded my surgical scrubs, I stuck my feet in a toilet and flushed it several times before removing my shoes. They eventually dried out, but I was glad to leave them behind when I finished the internship.

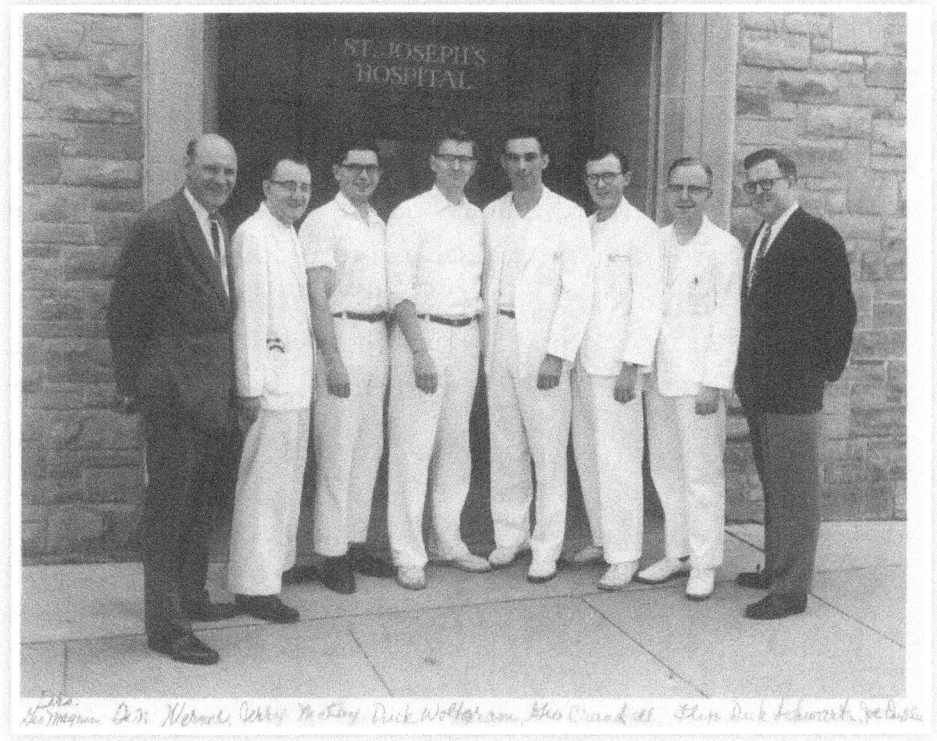

Interns

OFF TO THE ARMY

When we finished our internships those of us who hadn't been in the service had two choices: we could enlist as captains in the medical corps or wait to be drafted as buck privates. I don't know of anyone who waited to be drafted. After I enlisted I was ordered to report to Ft. Sam Houston in Texas for basic training. Compared to normal basic training ours was like a Sunday school picnic, in fact my two years in the army were more of a long vacation compared to my grueling internship.

In the morning and at noon we would fall in for formation then march off to our classes, accompanied by music from an army band to keep us in step. Most days consisted entirely of lectures but we had two days at a rural camp where we learned to fire various weapons, throw grenades and crawl under live machine gun fire. Every day at five o'clock we would all go home. We found a comfortable place to live at an old motel north of town which had a swimming pool. It was a great luxury to be able to go home every night, have a swim and make friends with our new neighbors.

PSYCHIATRIC TRAINING

In about the sixth week of our eight week training, a bird colonel named Cameron told our class that six of us could volunteer for on-the-job training in psychiatry and remain at Ft. Sam Houston for another twelve weeks. He assured us that those of us who were married would not be sent to Korea but would be stationed at a major army post in the states. I was married and had an infant daughter, and I really didn't want to go to Korea, so I promptly volunteered. The war in Korea was over by then, but I still didn't want to be away from my family for two years.

Our training took place in a locked psychiatric building which was part of Brooke Army Hospital. It consisted mostly of case presentations and interpretations by our chief instructor, another bird Colonel. We were each assigned patients and instructed to give them huge doses of Thorazine which was about the only anti-psychotic drug available then. We also were taught to administer insulin shock, Pentothal (truth serum) interviews and electroshock therapy (EST). The latter was a pretty brutal procedure which consisted of strapping electrodes to the patient's head and connecting them to an electrical current until the patient started having grand mal seizures. Someone had once observed that epileptics don't go crazy and assumed that the convulsions had something to do with it, so we gave them convulsions. That always produced profound retrograde amnesia. The patients wouldn't know where they were or what had happened to them, but they knew they didn't like it. In many cases two treatments would cause the patient to say "Hey, I'm fine now. I'm ready to go back to duty. I don't need any more treatments". EST is still used today, mostly for depression in which it has some success. In the rare case in which it is used, the patient is first anesthetized to avoid compression fractures of the spine, which sometimes occurred the way we did it

Some of our patients were simply goof-offs who couldn't or wouldn't adjust to army life, but some of them really were crazy. Probably the most important thing we learned was how to tell the difference. At the end of our training, true to the colonel's word, I was assigned to Fort Riley, Kansas, not to Korea

FORT RILEY

As "Division Psychiatrist" for the First Infantry Division I was stationed at the Mental Health Clinic, a small wooden barracks building, under the tutelage of Major Larry McGonagle, a real psychiatrist, along with Lt. Marvin West, a social worker, and

Lt. Paul Singer, a PhD psychologist. We also had five or six tech specialists, a regular army sergeant and two typist privates. Our mornings were spent dealing with referrals, mostly from company commanders, and our afternoons doing "psychotherapy" with selected army personnel and dependents. The First Infantry Division was still receiving draftees for basic training, and a lot of our work consisted of boarding people out of the army under the provisions of Army Regulations 635-208 (undesirable) and 635-209 (unsuitable). We also saw some soldiers who were just crazy, i.e. insane, and usually sent them to the psychiatric ward at the hospital. Twice a week we went to the post stockade where we did pretty much the same thing with newly admitted prisoners. Larry McGonagle, Marv West and Paul Singer were all wonderful people and a pleasure to work with. After about a month I became comfortable with my new work, which actually involved very little effort.

PRIVATE KOHN

The most skillful practitioner of passive-aggressive behavior I ever met was Hyman Kohn, a draftee from New York City. His main aim in life seemed to be to infuriate people, not by what he did but by what he didn't do, and he was really good at it. He could even salute in a way that was insolent and insulting. He was sent to me to see if he was competent to stand trial for refusing to obey a direct order, that being to shave off his curly black beard. He offered no excuse for not shaving, he just wouldn't do it. Army officers are not accustomed to being thwarted by buck privates, and his company commander was clearly furious with him. His past history revealed typical passive-aggressive personality disorder and no reason why he shouldn't stand trial. I recommended that he be boarded out as unsuitable, but his company commander really wanted him to be punished.

I attended his court martial to see what would happen. His defense counsel presented the argument that many famous army officers in the past had beards, but, as I expected, his body language and refusal to use the word "sir" had infuriated the six man court within half an hour. When he was found guilty and the court adjourned, Pvt. Kohn refused to salute the President of the Court, a full colonel. Six officers were screaming at him to salute, but he wouldn't, and there was nothing they could do about it. He was finally hauled off to the stockade to await sentencing. In the stockade he still refused to shave and was driving everyone crazy because they couldn't make him do it. By this time his case was well known all over the post and finally came to the attention of the commanding general who wisely said "I want that man off this post and out of the army before sundown". Three star generals usually get what they want, and that was the last I heard of Private Kohn.

COYOTES AND A HOOT OWL

An interesting case involved a staff sergeant whom a farmer allegedly observed regularly having intercourse with two dead coyotes and a hoot owl on his farm. The most interesting thing was that the MPs had built an elaborate blind equipped with movie cameras to film him in the act. I was required to watch the movies which confirmed the allegations. They showed the sergeant, in full color and in broad daylight, having intercourse with the coyotes and owl which the farmer had shot and hung on a fence. I didn't know of any regulations dealing with buggering coyotes, dead or alive, let alone hoot owls, so I passed the buck by sending him to the psychiatric ward at the hospital. I don't remember what happened to him , but I'm sure he was boarded out of the service. The sergeant had a wife and three children.

COLLEGE BASKETBALL STAR

One day I was called to the Colonel's office and told that a staff car was waiting to take me to the Riley County Hospital in nearby Manhattan, Kansas where I was to report to a certain local doctor. When I arrived there and contacted the doctor he explained the situation. One of his patients was a star on the Kansas State basketball team who roomed in the home of a young married couple. He and the wife had been having a clandestine affair, and the wife told him that day that it had to stop. The young man told the wife that he couldn't live without her and threatened to kill her. She called the police who arrested him and, at his request, called the doctor. He was released to the doctor's custody (first mistake) and admitted to a regular private room in the hospital (second mistake) where he went completely wild. He smashed furniture, broke glasses and threatened to kill the doctor. He also ate some of the broken glass fragments. When the doctor tried to subdue him he hit the doctor on the head with the leg of a broken chair. The doctor called the police again. The usual procedure in such cases is for two men to hold mattresses in front of them and crowd the patient into a corner where he could be subdued, but this was a very tall young man who simply reached over the mattresses and smashed his attackers on the head with the broken chair leg. I guess they never thought of football helmets and shoulder pads, and they abandoned the effort (third mistake). The patient was clearly in a murderous rage, and everyone was afraid of him. The doctor was considering telling the police to shoot him in the legs, and they might have done it.

I had no idea what the doctor expected me to do, but I didn't have sense enough to ask him. When I was shown to the patient's room I found the hallway absolutely full of yelling people, including a priest who was talking through the door with the patient. Because of the patient's fame as a basketball player the local newsmen were on hand with a great many questions for me. I guess an army psychiatrist was supposed to have answers. I didn't. My first instruction was to barricade the door, which had no lock, and get everyone out of the hall except for one person to silently observe him through the door's small window. I thought if all the attention was withdrawn he would eventually calm down, and that proved to be the case. After about half an hour he called for the doctor and allowed him to administer a powerful sedative The police put him in hand cuffs and hauled him off to jail, then the staff car took me back to the post where I retrieved my car and went home. It was a completely stupid but interesting day.

THE LORD'S PRAYER ON A GRAIN OF RICE

One day a middle aged soldier was sent to me because he claimed to be able to print the Lord's Prayer on a grain of rice and thus was assumed to be insane. In the course of the interview he produced several grains of rice from his pocket and asked me to inspect them with a magnifying glass. When I did that I could see that each grain did indeed have the Lord's Prayer printed on it. He refused to tell me how he did that, saying that it was a trade secret. I kept one of the grains and carried it for several years before I lost it somewhere. I still have no idea how he did it.

ACUTE LYMPHOCYTIC CHORIOMENINGITIS

About once every six weeks each of us medical officers was required to cover the emergency room and spend the night at the army hospital to deal with whatever came up. None of us liked that, but it was a chance for me to be a regular doctor instead of a psychiatrist. There was always a large number of soldiers and dependents to be seen in the emergency room, a few of whom were severely sick or injured. On one such occasion I saw a corporal with a headache, fever and stiff neck. I did a spinal tap and found a large number of lymphocytes but no bacteria in his spinal fluid. As an intern I had seen such a case and was told that it was acute lymphocytic choriomeningitis, a self limited disease. I assumed that it was fairly common, and that was my diagnosis. I know now that it could have been several other things, but, through sheer luck, it turned out that I was right. I have never seen or heard of another case since then.

The doctor who did the overnight duty wore a leather badge bearing the letters MOD for "Medical Officer of the Day". Protocol dictated that the MOD would return the badge to the hospital commander the following morning and give a brief report. The commander was an old colonel and not very well respected. Some of the MODs would just throw the badge on his desk and leave, but I always gave him a smart salute and a respectful report. He was very impressed with my diagnosis of ALC and astutely observed that it was a mouse borne disease. My respectful behavior was probably responsible for his awarding me an official commendation when I was discharged from the army.

DAYTON, OHIO

My agreement with the Illinois Agricultural Association allowed me to have another year of training before I had to start general practice in a small Illinois town. I wanted more training in surgery, so I wrote to three or four surgical residencies during my last year in the army. I visited the one at Good Samaritan Hospital in Dayton and decided to go there. After my discharge in June, 1958, the army moved my few belongings and my family to Dayton. I now had a two year old daughter and a one year old son.

I had always been good at making friends and adjusting to new situations, and I expected to do that in Dayton. I was surprised to discover that I was one of only two Americans on the house staff of about sixty. Most were Asians or Middle Easterners along with a few Germans, and they tended to associate with their countrymen and avoid others. Whereas I had three congenial surgical instructors in Marshfield, I had about fifteen at Good Samaritan, and they tended to ignore me. My immediate supervisor was the only other surgical resident, a Mexican martinet who called me Ervin and insisted that I call him Dr. Rodriguez. After about six weeks I had made no friends and was very unhappy. So was my wife. I also didn't care much for Dayton, which was a large, unfriendly city. I'm sorry to admit that I just couldn't handle the sudden comedown from army life, and I became very depressed. Although it was against my principles, I decided to resign from the residency and start a practice in Illinois.

WARMOLTS CLINIC

My family and I temporarily moved in with my in-laws in Geneva, Illinois, a small town west of Chicago, while I looked for a place to open a practice. I visited doctors in eight small towns to get a feel for the local situation. They were all fairly cordial, but not very interested in increasing the local doctor supply. The one exception was Lambertus Warmolts MD in Oregon, Illinois. He was about seventy and was the sole owner of the town's hospital. He was a Fellow of the American College of Surgeons, and his hospital was accredited by the JCAH, which was unusual for a small town hospital. He was a very charismatic old man and said he would be happy to have me work with him and learn to do more surgery.

I rented a house in town, but it wouldn't be available for three weeks, so I spent the first three weeks living in a room in the basement of the hospital and going back to Geneva on the weekends. Also living in the basement were his spooky scrub nurse Ethyl, his very obese bookkeeper Blanche, and his German janitor Charley.

Dr. Warmolts was a slender, burr-cut old man who water skied on the nearby Rock river every day from May through September. He owned three vehicles: an old, one seat Plymouth business coupe which he drove most of the time, a Cadillac sedan which he used to transport Ethyl and Blanche, and a Mercedes 300 SL sports car, cream colored with red leather upholstery. The 300 SL was known as the "gull wing" Mercedes because its doors were hinged at the top and resembled the wings of a gull when they were open. He claimed to have worn out three airplanes flying back and forth to Chicago. He also owned a 30 foot sailing sloop which he kept on lake Ponchartrain in Louisiana. He lived alone in a large house a little south of town on the Rock river.

I worked for Dr. Warmolts (for $700/month) for about a year and mostly learned what not to do by watching his failures. He had done some surgical training in Vienna in the thirties and hadn't changed a thing since then. Our only anesthesia was open drop ether administered by a poorly trained nurse. Ether is a very safe anesthetic, but it can be lethal if it isn't used right. It's also very unpleasant to inhale and usually produces severe nausea when the patient wakes up. Thinking it would be safer,

I persuaded Dr. Warmolts to let me use spinal anesthesia whenever I could. I'd had no training in its use, but I bought a book about it and had good luck with it.

I finally realized that we were practicing substandard medicine and decided to open an independent practice in town, which made him very angry. It was a very pretty little town on the Rock River about 50 miles west of Chicago. I had acquired a small following and a few friends and didn't want to move again. I was accepted on the staff of hospitals in Rockford, Dixon and Rochelle and opened an office above one of the town's two drug stores. I soon realized that having patients in all three hospitals would require most of the day just to make rounds, and limited my admissions to Rochelle. That was a 25 bed, modern hospital with a congenial medical staff of about seven other doctors. It was about twenty miles east of Oregon.

In addition to Warmolts, who didn't see many patients, there were three other doctors in town. Bob Catey had an office in the hospital and shared in its profits. Ray Mann looked and acted a lot like Lawrence Welk. Warmolts hated him but tolerated him because he admitted patients to the hospital. Frank Swann had an office over the other drug store and used the hospital in Dixon. Frank was the most competent of the three, and we got along well.

TOILET DELIVERY

One evening I answered the phone and the following exchange took place:

"Doc, it's George, my wife's having her baby. Hurry."

Me: "Wait, wait George. Where do you live?"

George: "Grand Detour, down by the river. Second house on the right."

Grand Detour was, fortunately, a very small settlement about eight miles south of town. When I finally located George's house, his wife had delivered her baby while sitting on the toilet but hadn't passed the placenta. George had fished the baby out of the toilet, and it was doing fine. I delivered the placenta and persuaded George to take mother and baby to the hospital in Rochelle for the customary five days of rest and observation. There were no complications.

MOVING ON

I had a marginally successful practice and a few friends in Oregon, but I didn't like practicing alone and felt that I wasn't making much progress. The town was very much controlled by its conservative, old aristocracy. After the bank turned down my application for a mortgage loan, I started to think about moving to a more hospitable town. In late 1959 I saw an ad in a medical journal from a former medical school friend and decided to investigate. The ad was an offer to join a three man group in Fairbury, a very small town in central Illinois, with a starting salary of $1,000/month, about $300 more than I was making. Fairbury turned out to be an old fashioned farm town with one main street. Most of the businesses still had high metal roofs over the sidewalk, so it looked like a town in an old western movie.

The medical group consisted of Drs. Henry Sauer, age 74, Bill Marshall, 72 and my friend Joe Novak. All were competent doctors and were very busy. I was most impressed by the town's 100 bed modern hospital. The town was not at all pretty and was surrounded by corn and soybean farms, most of which were owned by members of the Apostolic Christian Church, a very liberal branch of the Amish. The situation felt right to me, and I decided to join the group. It turned out to be a good decision.

FAIRBURY

After about six months I also became very busy. My partners were very congenial, and, with their help, I was starting to feel competent with surgical procedures. We had offices in a storefront in Fairbury and in an old building in the nearby town of Forrest. I had office hours in both towns. There were a lot of young people in Fairbury, and I soon had many friends. There were six other doctors on the hospital's medical staff: two in Fairbury and four in small towns east of there. We all got along well and spent a lot of time in each others homes.

One of my first house calls was to an elderly couple who lived in a house trailer. I don't remember why I was called there, but I found that the wife had very dry skin, dry, thinning hair, a puffy face and other signs of hypothyroidism. I drew some blood and sent it off for a protein bound iodine test, which was the best test then for hypothyroidism. It confirmed my diagnosis, so I started her on gradually increasing doses of thyroid. In a short time she showed remarkable improvement. Her two daughters were prominent in the community, and my reputation was soon spread widely.

Within a year I was an extremely busy doctor. I usually saw 20-25 patients each day in the office, made 3-5 house calls and each week did 2-3 major surgeries and 3-5 minors. I delivered around 80 babies every year (until the advent of birth control pills cut that way down) and usually had 15-20 patients in the hospital at any given time. That required working about 80 hours every week. It was unusual to sleep through the night without having to make a house call or go to the hospital at least once.

DRS. SAUER AND MARSHALL

Henry C. Sauer and William A. Marshall had both been practicing in Fairbury for many years before I arrived. Dr. Sauer was still doing a lot of surgery when I joined the group, but started to slow down soon after that. He was a good doctor and tried hard to keep up with modern medicine.

Dr. Marshall was born and educated in Canada and was, I think, a doctor in the RCAF during World War I. I don't know when or why he came to Fairbury. He could rightly be described as "sprightly". He had very erect posture and was usually very cheerful.

DRS. LANGSTAF AND MOSCICKI

The other two doctors in town, besides our group, were Jim Langstaff and Lucjan Moscicki. Jim's father had been a doctor who practiced in Fairbury for many years until his death. Jim had a farm east of town where he kept several horses and a very nice airplane.

Lucjan Moscicki was born in Poland and was in the Polish army during WW II. He was captured by the Russians and sent to Siberia, but he somehow escaped and walked out through the Caucasus to Palestine where he became attached to the British Eighth Army. After the war he went to medical school in Italy where he either met or renewed acquaintance with his wife, Christina, who had been some kind of Polish royalty before the war and had been active in the underground resistance. She also went to medical school but never repeated her internship in the US as foreign graduates are required to do. We became good friends. In about 1962 Lucjan's younger sister emigrated to the US and lived with his family. After about two weeks he sent her to live with my family for a month because he said she would never learn English at his house where they spoke Polish. She did learn quickly with us and later graduated from the University of Illinois.

OUR NEW OFFICE

My partners had already planned to build us a new office building, which they could well afford. It was a beautiful, well-designed building, and it improved our efficiency considerably. We went from three examining rooms to eight and had a well equipped lab, X-ray, minor surgery and pharmacy. There was a phone in every examining room because we had to be readily available to the hospital and because we thought we should personally respond to urgent calls. Our front office person could direct urgent incoming calls to whichever room we were in.

MEDICATIONS

Like most country doctors, we dispensed our own medications, which was a great help to our bottom line and an annoyance to the owner of the local drug store. As well as being a convenience for our patients it saved them some money since we only marked up the prices 20% above our cost. The person who filled our prescriptions was a housewife who had no training beyond high school. That may have been illegal, but she had been doing it for years and never made a mistake that I knew of.

The older doctors believed in preserving some of the mystery about the practice of medicine and had for years used a numeric code to identify medications. They would order meds using this code, and it would be written on the box or bottle given to the patient. It was common for patients to come in and say "I need another box of 409s" for example. I didn't want to bother learning the code, and I thought it was an unnecessary possible source of errors. I also thought that people should know what they were taking, so I ordered drugs by name and had the name written on the box. To their credit, the older doctors quit using their numeric code.

Both of our offices had an entry vestibule which was left unlocked and had a little box on the wall where we would leave prescriptions to be picked up after hours. We always got a lot of calls after hours, many of which could be dealt with over the phone. To avoid the need for going to the office to get medications I conceived the idea of leaving a small amount of the most commonly needed ones in coded packages in the vestibule boxes. We could then tell the patient to go and pick up a coded package and avoid the need to leave home and charge for an office call. They were often puzzled about how I knew to put that package out before they even called. That system worked very well until someone, probably the owner of the local drugstore, reported it to the state authorities. I was called to Springfield and instructed to stop doing it or lose my license. I reluctantly stopped.

ATTEMPTED SUICIDE

When we moved into our new building we hired a full time lab/X-ray technician, Red Watson. He was a good- natured, conscientious man who was a licensed mortician, but he hadn't practiced that profession for a long time. Instead he had been a lab/X-ray tech at the hospital. There was no computerized lab or X-ray equipment then; everything was done by hand.

I don't recall why a young married woman from Forrest came to see me, but I remember being puzzled by her story and ordering some blood work. After she had left Red accidentally dropped and broke the vial containing her blood and had to call her to apologize and ask her to return so he could draw more blood. Later that afternoon she was brought to the hospital unconscious having tried to kill herself with sleeping pills. Fortunately she didn't have enough pills to be fatal. When she regained consciousness she confided in me that she had recently had an affair with an itinerant truck driver and was afraid she had contracted a venereal disease. When Red asked her to come back for more blood work she assumed that we had found evidence of VD and knew that she would be exposed. I told her that Red really had dropped and broken the tube and that there was no evidence of VD. She asked me if she should confess to her husband, and I advised her to talk with a minister about that.

THE "AMISH"

Probably half of the community belonged to the Apostolic Christian church or had parents or grandparents who did. They were called "Amish", but they were not "horse and buggy Amish". They drove cars, used modern farm equipment and had modern ideas about business and politics. They were, on the whole, friendly, honest people and good farmers and business men. They were mostly of German descent. In addition to one Catholic church and several Protestant churches, there were two Amish churches in town. The "brick church" was the oldest and most conservative. Its members wore pretty typical Amish attire. They didn't support formal education or birth control and tended to have large families. The "white church", which was in a large wooden building painted white, was more liberal. Its members wore normal clothes, and I think some of their children went to college. I don't think either church had a steeple or a bell or a paid minister.

It was common for Amish children to get a little wild in their late teens while they decided whether or not to "join church". It seemed that those who decided not to join were not censured in any way. It appeared to be completely voluntary.

We hear stories about country doctors being paid with baked goods and produce, and our Amish patients did sometimes bring us such things, but they also paid their bills.

GLENN HUDGENS, MD

About half way through my third year in Fairbury, Joe Novak left to become the medical director of an insurance company in Chicago. That left me having to deal with his practice as well as mine. In the following nine months I had only three days off, when I was able to persuade him to briefly come back and cover for me. That was a very hard nine months.

After a lot of effort, I was finally able to recruit a new partner, Glenn Hudgens, who had just finished his internship. He was a great partner and a wonderful person. After he had been with us for about ten days, I left for a ten day vacation. It was a cruel thing to do, but he endured it. We subsequently practiced together for eight years, during which he also became a good surgeon.

Glenn had a great sense of humor and was usually very support-ive of me. He was a good doctor, and the patients loved him.

TWINS AND TRIPLETS

One of our occasional visiting specialists was a neurosurgeon named David Moore. He was born in Fairbury but practiced neurosurgery with his uncle in Chicago. During one of his rare visits he told me that he and his wife had been trying, without success, to start a family for a long time and that about a year ago, they decided to adopt. They fell in love with a pair of twins in an orphanage and adopted them. Within a short time, his wife became pregnant and ultimately delivered triplets, and they now had five babies in diapers. This story has nothing to do with me, but I thought it was interesting.

"THERE ARE DIRECTIONS IN THE BOX"

During the months before Glenn Hudgens arrived, I was called to the hospital to deal with the multiple victims of a horrible auto accident which had occurred just west of town. A man and his wife, baby, mother-in-law and father-in-law had been in a car which collided head-on with a large Oldsmobile driven by a single woman. The wife was dead when I arrived. The father had a broken arm, and the baby was leaking spinal fluid from one ear, indicating a skull fracture, but was otherwise unhurt. The mother-in-law had a head injury and was unconscious. The father-in-law, had no apparent injuries. The other driver, the single woman, had multiple injuries. Her nose and face were smashed, and her right eye was lying on her cheek. There were no breath sounds in her right lung, and her right hip appeared to be dislocated. Her airway was severely compromised, so I did an emergency tracheotomy. I put her eye back in its socket and covered it with a vaseline dressing, then I packed her bleeding nose. While she was in X-ray, I put the baby on antibiotics and called one of my older partners to deal with the man with the broken arm. X-rays revealed that the single woman did have a dislocated hip and a right hemo-pneumothorax, i.e.the lung was collapsed and bleeding. Also, her third cervical vertebra was fractured. Miraculously, the spinal cord wasn't damaged. When I saw that fractured vertebra, I almost had an involuntary bowel movement. I had extended her neck to do the tracheotomy!

I put two chest tubes in the woman's chest, put her right leg in traction and called David Moore to ask for help with the unconscious woman, the baby with a fractured skull and the woman with a broken neck. David said that he had two surgeries scheduled the next morning and couldn't come. He said I should just observe the baby, pack the unconscious woman in ice and put Crutchfield tongs in the other woman's skull. He said that we had them in our surgical supplies. I told him that I didn't know how to do that, and he said there were directions in the box. Crutchfield tongs are used to apply traction to the skull and spine. They are like small ice tongs. To use them, one bores two holes in the top of the skull, inserts the tongs and tightens a screw to clamp the tongs together. I did what the directions said and applied traction to the tongs to prevent damage to the spinal cord.

The unconscious mother-in-law died during the night. I don't know if she could have been saved, but there was nothing I could do. The father and baby recovered and were discharged. After a few days the other woman's hip came back into place, and her lung re-inflated and stopped bleeding. I removed the chest tubes and leg traction and sent her, by ambulance, to David in Chicago.

I saw that woman a few months later in my office. Her neck had healed; her nose had been fixed, and she had a prostheses in place of her right eye. I found out that she was a barbiturate addict and had been "high" at the time of the accident. A month or so later, I was called to Springfield to testify at a trial concerning her. After explaining all the details, I was asked what my fee had been for taking care of her. It was $300. Even at that time, it should have been $1,000, but our fees were modest. One of my friends who is still in practice says that today it would probably be about $200,000.

ENDTABLE DEATH TRAP

One of my patients was an elderly, short, chubby lady who was living alone since the recent death of her husband. Her daughter asked me to go to her house to see why she wouldn't answer her phone. I still don't know why the daughter didn't go herself or why I agreed to do it, but I did. No one locked their doors in that community, and I just walked in when she failed to answer my knock. There was a couch in her living room with a glass topped end table at each end. I found the lady dead with her arms and legs sticking out of the top of one of the end tables. Something had caused her to sit on it which broke the glass, and she fell into it, bottom first. She was trapped. Maybe she stumbled or had a stroke or fainted. I didn't know how long she had been there, but I hate to think what her last minutes or hours must have been like.

"I CUT ELMER A LITLE"

Elmer and Blanche had been married for several years, and they argued a lot. One evening Blanche called, and this exchange followed:

Blanche: Doc, it's Blanche. Come over.

Me: What for?

Blanche: You just come.

Me: Dammit Blanche, you're always doing this. You have to tell me why.

Blanche: I cut Elmer a little.

Me: Let me talk to Elmer.

Blanche: He can't talk.

Me: Why not?

Blanche: He's laying here on the floor.

Me: I'll be there in five minutes.

When I arrived, I found Elmer on the kitchen floor with a wound through his left arm and a sucking wound in his chest. A butcher knife was on the floor. He had obviously thrown up his arm to protect himself before Blanche stabbed him. When I got him to the hospital, I put in a chest tube to re-inflate his lung and repaired the wound in his arm. He recovered in a few days and went home. He refused to press charges against Blanche, and they resumed their quarrelsome married life.

SNOW STORM

It seemed to me that everyone in the large Mortz family was a little nutty. I got a call in the middle of a winter night from a Mortz who lived on a farm west of town asking me to come to his house because one of his children wasn't breathing. A blizzard was raging outside, and the snow was at least two feet deep. I said my car wouldn't get me there, but he insisted that I try so I did. I got completely stuck about a half mile from his house and set off on foot carrying my bag. In about ten minutes a jeep came along and took me the rest of the way. I found the parents and some neighbors drinking coffee in the kitchen. When I asked to see the child, his father said "Oh he's fine now. I was wrong". The man with the jeep took me home, and I had a wrecker recover my car the next morning. I charged eight dollars for that call, and Mortz protested that the charge was excessive. A typical Mortz.

NOTHING WRONG WITH CHARLIE

I often made hospital rounds with one or two of my partners. On one occasion three of us stopped to see one of Dr. Sauer's elderly patients who was a known hypochondriac. Dr. Sauer said "There's really nothing wrong with Charlie here". At that moment Charlie died, right in front of us, as if to say "I'll show you". Dr. Sauer was at a loss for words. My other partner and I left him to deal with the situation and went on about our rounds.

MARFAN'S AND EHLERS-DANLOS

One of my early patients had Marfan's syndrome, a very rare condition characterized by a very tall, lean frame, long, narrow fingers, an abnormality of the ocular lens and an abnormality of the aorta. She suddenly died sitting in my waiting room. I had been prescribing Quinidine to treat her rapid heart rate, and that may or may not have been what killed her. I had recently read a journal article about closed-chest cardiac massage, and I tried that, but to no avail. Her sister, an OB nurse, had Ehlers-Danlos syndrome, an also very rare condition characterized by weak, rubbery ligaments. Her feet were absolutely flat, and all of her joints were floppy. It had no known relation to Marfan's. Having two sisters with very rare, unrelated conditions was extremely unusual, but I never investigated further. Maybe I should have. These conditions did have some features in common and may someday be shown to be genetically related.

HERMAN WELMERLING

In the early years, our most frequent visiting specialist was Dr. Herman Welmerling from Bloomington. During World War Two, Bloomington was left with no orthopedists or urologists. Dr. Welmerling filled the gap by becoming a self-made combination orthopedist/urologist. I don't know how he did it, but he was pretty competent. He did all of our hip pinnings and transurethral prostate resections. He was about sixty years old. He also helped with complex fractures, often using a method called external fixation, which was developed by a veterinarian named Stader. They were called Stader Splints and involved putting pins into bones through the skin and aligning them with an external device like an erector set. The method had fallen into disrepute, but he had pretty good luck with it.

FISHING FOR STONE

Our group allowed each of us to take two weeks off for postgraduate study every year. I usually spent those two weeks at the Cook County Graduate School of Medicine in Chicago taking advanced courses in surgery, obstetrics, ear nose and throat, etc. They involved lectures, demonstrations and hands-on experience at the Cook County Hospital. We often had to call Dr. Welmerling to do cystoscopies and retrograde pyelograms, so I took a two week course in urology and learned to do those procedures. I also learned how to use a Vermier Basket to pull a stone out of a ureter in certain circumstances. I only had occasion to use a Vermier Basket once, and it was successful. It was more fun than catching a big fish!

OBSTETRIC RECTALS

Up until the mid sixties it was standard practice to check the stage of an OB patient's dilation through the rectum to reduce the risk of postpartum sepsis. In about '63 I took a 2 week course in OB at the Cook County Hospital and was taught that one could safely check dilation vaginally using a sterile glove. When I did that with my next OB patient the nurse was horrified, but I assured her that it was perfectly safe As luck would have it, the patient developed a roaring case of postpartum endometritis. Fortunately that was the last case I ever saw.

VERSION AND EXTRACTION

When one of my OB patients was having a prolonged labor I discovered that she had a "shoulder presentation", i.e. the baby's shoulder was in the birth canal instead of the head. This, of course, is an impossible delivery. There are two possible courses of action: You can do a Caesarian section or what is called a version and extraction. This latter maneuver involves grasping the baby's heel and pulling it out by the foot, which is nowhere near as simple as it sounds and is, in fact, very dangerous. In addition to the dangers of a breech delivery, which are considerable, one runs the risk of rupturing the uterus or getting hold of a hand instead of a foot which would only compound the problem.

It was around two A.M. The mother was exhausted, and I was too. It would take at least an hour to get a surgical team and anesthesia in place, and , in those days, a C Section had significant risks of its own. In between contractions her uterus became very relaxed. When I reached into it, I thought I could feel a heel, and I succumbed to the temptation. I told the OB nurse to anesthetize the patient with open drop ether, which she did. When I was sure I had hold of a heel, I started gently pulling on it and continued until the baby was turned around into a breech position, then stopped the anesthesia. With the help of a few contractions I was able to deliver the baby. Once again, I was a very lucky doctor. A very, very lucky doctor.

ANSWERING MACHINES

In about 1965 Glenn and I both got rudimentary telephone answering machines. They wouldn't take messages, but they would answer calls by saying who was on call. For the first time we were not both constantly on call. When I got home on my night or weekend off I would turn on the machine before I even took my coat off. It was a huge relief, and I loved it, but my friends and relatives hated "that damned machine".

DON L. ERVIN, MD

CARNIVAL WOMAN DEODORIZED

The Livingston County fair was held in Pontiac, the county seat, but Fairbury had its own fairgrounds and annual fair, including a carnival. The carnival people almost seemed to save up their problems until they got to Fairbury where they knew we would take care of them, almost always for no compensation. Four of us local doctors rotated call for unattached patients in the ER on a weekly basis. We all dreaded being on call during Fair week.

I was "it" when a woman and her boyfriend from the carnival brought in the woman's elderly mother with second degree burns on her forearms and thighs. I learned that she had, for some weeks, been living in the back seat of the boyfriend's old Buick. If she tried to get out to relieve herself, it was obvious that she didn't always make it in time. She was the filthiest, smelliest live person I had ever seen. Agnes Runyon, an ex-army nurse, had ER duty that night. She was a pretty tough lady, but she vomited in a floor bucket about halfway through my exam. I barely avoided that myself. After we cleaned and dressed the woman's burns, I admitted her for observation and a clean-up.

When I saw the woman the next morning, the change was remarkable. The nurses had thoroughly bathed her and had her in a fresh hospital gown, and her beautiful white hair was tied up with a blue ribbon. I discharged her after a day or so, and she probably returned to her den in the old Buick.

PACGC

Some patients exaggerate the severity of their symptoms, and this is usually obvious to an experienced physician. Sometimes in such cases I prescribed PACGC, which was simply APC (asprin, phenacitin and caffine) but in green capsules instead of white tablets. I would caution them to use them sparingly because they were "very strong". They usually found them very helpful.

HAND AMPUTATION

One of our local industries was the Honegger Corporation which had a big egg operation in Forrest and a bulk blending plant in Fairbury where various grains were mixed into livestock feed. One night I was called to the blending plant where an employee had got his left hand and wrist into a corn grinder. With a few wrenches I was able to dismantle the machine enough to extract what remained of his hand which resembled a bag full of dice. When bones, nerves and vessels are all damaged there was, at that time, no choice but to amputate. We got him medicated and to the hospital where I amputated his left hand above the wrist, and he had an uneventful recovery. That was the only major amputation I ever did. My great grandfather did hundreds while he was a surgeon in the Civil War. He told my Dad that they ran out of chloroform during the invasion of Atlanta, and he had to do amputations with no anesthesia.

DON L. ERVIN, MD

INOVATIVE TREATMENT OF TIBIAL FRACTURE

Auto races were another fairground event, including midget racers each year. They attracted some big name drivers and made a lot of noise. One night the flag waver, who stands very near the speeding cars, stood too close and was brought in with a comminuted fracture of his tibia, the big bone in the lower leg, i.e. it was broken in three places. There are no significant nerves or vessels on either side of the anterior tibial tubercle (the knob below the knee) or the calcaneus (the heel bone), and one can insert pins through these places with little danger. After we anesthetised the patient and cleaned up his leg, I put a Rush pin through his anterior tibial tubercle and another through his calcaneus. Then I put a U shaped clamp on the lower pin and tied a rope from it to the steam radiator in the operating room. I had the anesthetist unlock the wheels on the operating table and pull back on it until the rope was very tight, then lock the wheels again. When X-ray confirmed that the bone fragments were well lined up, I enveloped the leg in plaster, incorporating the two pins. The bone healed nicely after several weeks and two cast changes. I should have just sent that patient to an orthopedic surgeon in Bloomington, but that option never occurred to me.

AN UNEXPECTED FINDING

In the fifties and sixties we didn't have all of the wonderful diagnostic aids that are available today. We relied a lot on physical findings. In medical school I was taught to do very thorough physical exams, and I continued to do that whenever possible.

Third stage syphilis effects mostly the heart and central nervous system. It often causes what is called an Argyll-Robertson pupil, i.e. one which will react to accommodation, contracting when the patient watches an object being moved closer, but will not react to light. This is a very subtle finding, but looking for it is part of a really thorough physical exam. We had almost no venereal disease in our community, but I continued to check eye signs out of habit.

Mrs. Rosenkrants, a respectable elderly lady who lived with her husband and 50 year old bachelor son, had a bad, recurrent ingrown toenail. I had operated on it twice, but it kept coming back. I finally decided to reduce the length of her toe and eliminate the nail altogether. This required admitting her to the hospital, and that required a complete physical exam. I was dumbfounded to find that she had an Argyll-Robertson pupil, but I finally saw what I had been missing for years. Her son had a caved-in looking nose, small, peg- shaped teeth and generally lax tissues. He was recently having trouble flexing his feet; all signs of congenital syphilis which he had acquired, in utero, from his mother. A serum test for syphilis was positive for the mother and son but negative for the husband. The disease had long since ceased to be contagious. I had to report this to the public health officials, but they were discrete, and nothing much was done about it. I knew nothing about Mrs. Rosenkrants's early history and decided that I didn't want to know. I treated both mother and son with penicillin which probably arrested the disease but didn't change much. I would <u>never</u> have suspected that Mrs. R had syphilis.

WART RUBBER

I had acquired some renown for my ability to rub warts with my thumb and make them go away. This, of course, was pure hocus pocus, but it often worked. If one rub didn't work, I would sometimes put the patient on the X-ray table and , cautioning them not to move, I would set the timer for five seconds. It made a clicking sound as it wound down. Of course I didn't turn on the X-ray, but that usually did the trick. I never charged for this service.

DUCK BONE PERFORATION

One evening a teenage boy was brought to the ER complaining of severe abdominal pain. His abdomen was rigid and exquisitely tender. He had no history of peptic ulcer, but an X-ray revealed air under the diaphragm indicating a perforated viscus, probably the stomach. When I opened his abdomen in the operating room, I found a two inch sliver of bone protruding from his stomach. I removed the bone, closed the hole and tacked some omentum over it. He later recalled eating some duck a few days earlier and having some trouble swallowing it. He somehow got that bone down his esophagus without perforating it, but it got stuck in his stomach. He made an uneventful recovery.

C.E. BRANCH, M.D.

Charlie Branch had practiced in Piper City since about 1936. It was a small town about 20 miles east of Fairbury. He and his partners, Hugh McIntosh and Harold Lockner, used our hospital. Charlie was a conscientious doctor and a good surgeon, and he helped me a few times when I had to do a procedure for the first time. We all had to deal with a lot of farm injuries, and one of his was especially unusual. The patient, a middle aged farmer, had stepped over the power takeoff on his tractor and caught the crotch of his pants in it. In a matter of seconds, it avulsed his scrotum, i.e. ripped it right off. The testicles were not damaged. Charlie repaired this injury with skin grafts, and, about a year later, the patient sired another child. I thought that was remarkable. Charlie died a few years ago at age 104.

ED AND PEARL

Ed and Pearl lived on a farm north of Fairbury. They had twenty one children, of which I delivered the last two. As part of my prenatal care, I usually gave the expectant mother a copy of a publication produced by the government which explained what to expect, what to eat, etc. As I was about to hand it to Pearl, I realized that she probably knew more about having babies than I or anyone in the government ever would, so I skipped that part. When I asked about her periods, she said that she hadn't had one since she was sixteen. She was always pregnant before the next one was due.

When Ed used his tractor there were usually several children riding on it with him. One day one of them fell off and into the manure spreader they were pulling. The child went partway through the blades of the spreader and had multiple, deep lacerations into which manure was ground. As I was trying to clean out and repair these lacerations, Ed said "I don't know Doc, I think it would be easier to make another one than to clean this one up". He actually said that to me.

DON'T FOOL WITH MOTHER NATURE

Betty Stark and her husband really wanted children but couldn't seem to have them. She had already had three spontaneous abortions (miscarriages) when she became pregnant again. In about the tenth week of her pregnancy she started showing signs of another miscarriage, and I was desperate to help her save this baby. I started giving her progesterone, and her bleeding stopped. After about two more months she again showed signs of an inevitable abortion, and I reluctantly did a D&C which yielded what is called a hydatidiform mole, not an undeveloped fetus. A hydatidiform mole is a grapelike cluster of cells derived from a pathological ovum which failed to abort at the usual time and sometimes leads to a chorionepithelioma which is a very malignant cancer of the uterus. I don't know how much my progesterone treatment had to do with that, but I clearly should not have done it. It was another case of unintended outcomes.

THE HOSPITAL

The Fairbury Hospital was a completely independent, modern, one hundred bed, nonprofit facility governed by a self-perpetuating board of volunteer directors. It received no tax support, and there were never any fund drives. It was probably organized as a 501 corporation so it could receive tax- deductible donations, and some people left sizable contributions to it in their wills. I don't know when or how it got started, but it was self-supporting all the time I was in Fairbury. Finding a modern hospital of that size in a town of about 2,500 people is extremely unusual, but we kept it full a good part of the time. Sometimes, in fact, we would have to discharge a patient before we could admit another one, and we would occasionally have to temporarily put a patient on a bed in the hall.

Up until Medicare was implemented the charge for a semi-private room was $16 per day. A private room was $18. No one was refused admission for lack of funds. We always had a very competent nursing staff, many of whom were LPNs. We never wanted for any kind of equipment, and we had a competent laboratory and X-ray department.

After I had been in town about seven years, our occupancy had decreased, and one of our three floors was closed. I'm not sure why. Probably our criteria for admission had gone up, or maybe we had already done most of the elective surgery needed by our population. In any case, the remaining floors kept busy.

About two years after I left town, Glenn moved to California. Harold Lockner had retired, and Charlie Branch was in the process. About ten years later, the hospital closed and was converted to a nursing home. I'm told that there is now only one doctor in town, a female.

THE SCHAEFERS

I took care of most of the large Schaefer family, including the grandfather, parents, children and grandchildren. I delivered one of the daughter's babies before I delivered her mother's last baby.

They were all quiet, gentle people who appreciated whatever I did for them. The grandfather complained frequently of headaches. When he developed a paralysis of the left side of his face, I assumed that it was Bell's palsy. I know now that it was probably an acoustic neuroma, but I didn't know anything about that at the time. I regret very much that I didn't. He was a really nice old man.

A RUN OF STILLBIRTHS

Altogether I delivered about eight hundred babies. Up until the mid sixties only two had been stillbirths, but then I had a run of six stillbirths out of the next ten consecutive deliveries. I had seen each of these women within a week before they went into labor and found no problems, but each of them had no fetal heart tones when they came to the hospital, indicating that their babies were dead. I have no idea why this happened, but it was very demoralizing. I only delivered one stillbirth after that group, and it was my fault. I still don't like to think about that one.

A SUCCESSFUL CLOSED-CHEST MASSAGE

In the middle of office hours, I got an emergency call from Huck Wilson saying that his wife was unconscious and gasping for breath. I rushed to their house, and she died as I entered her bedroom. She had no pulse and no heart sounds. I tried closed-chest resuscitation, and her heart started again, but she had very low blood pressure. When we got her to the hospital, I started an IV infusion of Levophed, a powerful vasoconstricor. I had used that drug before in extreme cases with limited success, and I almost thought of it as "the kiss of death", but it worked in this one. Her pressure came up, and we slowly weaned her off the drug. She recovered from her heart attack in a few weeks and went on to live for several years.

SEMIAUTOMATIC HISTORY AND PHYSICAL

Our hospital was very well equipped and well run, and I thought it could be accredited by the Joint Commission except for one thing. The other doctors had, for many years, kept very skimpy medical records, and the Joint Commission required a complete history and physical on every patient admitted. No one but me seemed to care much about accreditation, and I knew that persuading them to do all that increased paper work would be nearly impossible. I conceived a plan in which the doctor would fill out a one page sheet listing the Chief Complaint and brief Present Illness; mark on a matrix of physical findings to indicate "normal", "abnormal" or "not examined" and list below it any abnormalities, then indicate an admitting diagnosis. The nurses would administer a questionnaire covering the past history, family history and review of systems. When all of this was delivered to the medical records office, the people there would convert it into a complete history and physical using an automatic typewriter to fill in the normal findings.

To the great credit of the older doctors, they agreed to this plan, and it was implemented. About a year later we requested an evaluation by the Joint Commission, and our hospital was accredited.

A NEW LIFE FOR
AN OLD MAN

John Summers, about age seventy eight, had a long history of peptic ulcer. The ulcer had probably burned out some years ago, but the outlet from his stomach was severely constricted by scar tissue. Despite a very limited diet, he often became obstructed, and we had to admit him for decompression with a nasogastric tube. He was very thin.

After a few such episodes, I decided that John needed a gastroenterostomy, i.e. a connection between his stomach and his small bowel to bypass the constriction. I had never done that procedure, but I felt confident that I could, so we took John to the operating room. The procedure went well with no complications, and he made a nice recovery.

When I saw John a few months later he had gained a lot of weight and had a big smile on his face. He said he could eat anything he wanted to.

ROBERT F. BORT, MD

In about 1964 we persuaded Bob Bort to join our practice. He had just finished two years on an indian reservation in northern Minnesota with the US Public Health Service. He was a very tall, slim, red headed man and a natural born piano player. He was also a pretty good doctor. His wife seemed to dislike me from the very outset, saying that I was a "horse and buggy doctor". I never understood that, and she never got over it. In some ways she was probably right. He was with us until 1970 when he left to do a psychiatry residency.

EXCHANGE TRANSFUSIONS

Mating of an Rh positive man with an Rh negative woman can produce an Rh positive fetus. Often after one such fetus the woman will develop Rh antibodies with the next one which can cause severe hemolytic anemia in the newborn with jaundice and degenerative changes in the brain called Kernicterus. This can sometimes be minimized by prenatal treatment of the mother with a globulin called RhoGAM which we did in such cases, but it sometimes occurs anyway. The treatment in such cases is to drain the blood of the fetus through the umbilical cord and replace it with O negative blood. This is done in small increments and is called an exchange transfusion. This is usually done by a pediatrician but, of course, we did that too. Progress is gauged by measuring the infant's bilirubin. One exchange will usually do it, but I had one case which required three. It made me very nervous, but it turned out alright.

I mention this mostly to point out the scope and extent of our practice. We were among the few GPs who did exchange transfusions, and I doubt if any do today. One might reasonably ask why we did all these things. I think there were several reasons: In the 1960s it was still common for GPs to do OB and some surgery. We did more surgery than most because it was expected in our community and because I, like my father, was very much a "do-it-yourself" kind of person. Also it was a convenience for our patients to get things done locally. Finally, that's just the kind of doctor I wanted to be.

FEE SCHEDULE

Some of our typical fees in the early sixties were as follows:

Office visit..$2

Hospital visit..$5

House call, day or night..$5

Emergency room visit..$10

Tracheotomy..$50

Exchange transfusion..$25

OB delivery..$100

C section..$200

Appendectomy..$100

Hysterectomy..$200

Hernia repair..$100

Cholecystectomy (gall bladder)....................................$200

T&A (tonsils and adenoids)..$50

In spite of these low fees we made fairly good incomes because we did a lot of work. We were already in the fifty percent income tax bracket which meant that we would have to pay half of any additional income to the government, so we weren't very motivated to raise our fees.

ANESTHESIA

In Fairbury our anesthesia was administered by Dr. Marshall. He used IV Pentothal, a fast acting barbiturate, for induction and an anesthesia machine for the ether. He had done it for many years and was very good at it, but he had no experience with endotracheal tubes or muscle relaxing agents, both of which had been around for some years. When Dr. Bob Bort joined our practice in about 1964, we immediately sent him to Chicago for a thirty day course in anesthesiology at the Cook County Hospital. He was pretty inept when he returned, but he did know how to put in endotracheal tubes and use muscle relaxers and other agents besides ether. After a few months he became very competent at providing anesthesia.

PLACENTA PREVIA

I made my share of mistakes, maybe more than my share. Some were serious, and a few were very serious. Among the latter was the case of a pregnant lady whom I suspected of having a placenta previa because she'd had an episode of significant spontaneous bleeding a few weeks before her due date. When she went into labor I had to determine whether or not she had a previa, i.e. a placenta which covered the inside of the cervix. Today that is easily done with ultrasound, but then it could only be done by feel. I had been taught that one should have the patient on the operating table, prepared and draped for a caeserian section with a surgical team and anesthesia available before feeling to see if something soft was in front of the head. We were a small town hospital without all those people readily available, and I thought that, rather than to go to all that trouble, I would just feel very gently. That was a very serious mistake!

As soon as I very gently touched where the head should have been, blood started shooting out of the vagina like water out of a hose. I started two IVs with large bore needles, running saline through one and Dextran (a somewhat effective blood substitute) through the other. We rushed the patient to the operating room and called for the surgical team and Dr. Bort for anesthesia. I also ordered several pints of O negative blood which would have to come from the blood bank in Peoria. By this time the patient was in hypovolemic shock, and I was nearly in shock myself. When everyone was assembled the patient stopped bleeding, and I decided to hold everything until we could get her blood pressure up, which took about half an hour. When her pressure was up to a reasonable level we went ahead with the C section, and both mother and baby survived. I was a very lucky and thoroughly shaken doctor.

MULTIPLE SURGERIES ON ONE PATIENT

One of my patients was a very stoic middle aged farm wife who had a femoral hernia. I suggested that we should repair it, but she refused. When she was bought in with severe abdominal pain I assumed that her hernia was incarcerated and took her to the operating room. I was fixated on that femoral hernia. When

I repaired it I found that it was not incarcerated and decided that she must have appendicitis. I always used a paramedian incision for appendectomies because I thought it was more anatomical than a McBurney incision and because it could be extended upward if something else was wrong. I did the appendectomy and found her appendix normal. When I explored the abdomen I found that she had a perforated ulcer. I extended the incision upward and repaired the perforation. She had no history of peptic ulcer, but, as I said, she was a very stoic woman. She got three operations at once.

CHARLIE

Charles G McCarthy has been my steadfast friend for fifty years. I first met him when I was called to his house because he was having severe abdominal pain. He was a very big, somewhat intimidating Illinois State Policeman, a few years younger than me. His signs and symptoms were typical of gallbladder disease. After relieving his pain I arranged for a cholecystogram, which confirmed the presence of gall stones, and told him we would have to remove his gallbladder. Before we could schedule that surgery he developed jaundice, indicating that his common bile duct had become obstructed by a stone and making the surgery urgent.

At the time Charlie didn't know that his would be only the second gallbladder I had ever done, but I knew what I was doing, as evidenced by his uneventful recovery. In the following weeks we became close friends and have remained so till this day.

He was an ordinary trooper for eleven years before he finally made corporal. After he once got off the bottom step of the ladder he advanced rapidly through sergeant and lieutenant to captain and ultimately retired as commander of the district in which he had started.

We had lot of good times together, sometimes hunting and fishing at my parents' resort in Wisconsin and often working on projects, usually my projects. He was very helpful in restoring the cabin on my ranch in Colorado, building fences, etc. He seldom asked for my help on his projects which, of course, I would have gladly provided.

He still has his genial personality and wonderful sense of humor, and it's always a pleasure to see him.

GASTRIC HEMORRHAGE

Chuck West, the local Oldsmobile dealer, was a good friend of mine. He was about my age and was built like a football player. One afternoon he was brought to the ER in a wheelchair. When I got there I found him very pale, cold and perspiring profusely. He fainted as we were talking, and I threw the wheelchair onto its rear wheels to get his head lower than his body. When he regained consciousness he said that he had been vomiting what looked like coffee grounds, a sure sign of gastric bleeding, and had been having a lot of heartburn. I started two IVs with large bore needles, running saline through one and Dextran through the other, and ordered several pints of O negative blood from the blood bank in Peoria.

When we got him into a room I put down a nasogastric tube and started irrigating his stomach with ice water in an effort to stop the bleeding. I stood by his bed for six hours irrigating his stomach and giving him vitamin K and everything else I could think of, including the blood when it finally arrived. Late that evening when I had about decided to take him to surgery the bleeding stopped. I had been very reluctant to anesthetize him when he was on the edge of going back into shock for fear it would kill him. A few days later we got an upper GI fluoroscopy and found no sign of peptic ulcer. His bleeding was from acute hemorrhagic gastritis. I couldn't have done anything about it surgically.

DREAM HOUSE

I've always had a penchant for fixing up old things instead of buying new ones. It isn't just because I'm frugal. Sometimes it costs as much to fix up an old thing as it would to buy a new one, especially if my labor is counted. Maybe it's because I was raised during the great depression. In any case, I keep doing it. My "dream house" is a case in point.

There was an old, square, two story farm house on the south edge of town on about three acres of land. There were several big old oak trees around the house and on the north acre. I thought it had great potential and had been trying to buy it for awhile. I finally succeeded and engaged Melvin Zimmerman, a local contractor, to remodel it and build on an addition. We put in new wiring, heating and plumbing, and added a big family room on the back with a laundry room, bath room and screened porch. We put a brick portico on the front with four two story white columns. It had a stable and white fenced pasture for my daughter's old horse. I designed every bit of it, and I thought it was beautiful. We moved in early in 1966, as I recall.

MRS. ZIMMERMAN'S MULTI-PATHOLOGY

Melvin's wife developed moderate abdominal pain and nausea and had a tender abdomen. It seemed like appendicitis, but it was very mild, and I decided to watch it for awhile. When it didn't improve after a few days, we took her to surgery. I found that her appendix was very inflamed and had adhered to a large ovarian cyst and had ruptured into the cyst. She also had an obvious sarcoma of the uterus. We removed her ovarian cyst and appendix and her uterus, and she had an uneventful recovery.

NEWBORN WITH LARYNGOMALACIA

One of the babies I delivered had trouble breathing because its larynx was very soft and would collapse like a wet soda straw when it inhaled. In desperation I did a tracheotomy on the baby which temporarily solved the problem, then referred it to an ENT specialist. I later read that it wasn't possible to tracheotomise a newborn, but that obviously wasn't true.

A SIMPLE BOWEL OBSTRUCTION

A young woman, one of triplets delivered by Dr. Sauer, presented with vomiting and a distended, painful abdomen. Her bowel sounds, high pitched, tinkling rushes, were typical of a small bowel obstruction This was confirmed by X-ray which showed several loops of distended small bowel, several of which had air-fluid levels. There are several possible causes for a small bowel obstruction, and I felt competent to deal with whatever it might be. When we opened her abdomen we found that it was the simplest of all, a so-called congenital band. In such a case a band of fibrous tissue, present since birth, has contracted and occluded the bowel. I have no idea why this happens, but it does. I snipped the band, and we closed her up. She had no further problems.

FLOYD WEAVER, MD

Floyd Weaver, a board certified general and vascular surgeon, moved to Pontiac in about 1967, having just finished his residency at the Hines VA hospital. He was a Mennonite and went to medical school late in life. He was a gentle, quiet, modest man and a very competent surgeon, and he was very willing to come to the Fairbury Hospital whenever we needed him. I didn't do vascular surgery and tried to avoid bowel surgery, and it was a great relief to have him available. He was a pleasure to work with.

We did a lot of surgery together in the years that followed, including carotid endarterectomies, a procedure for removing obstructions in the carotid artery. This prevented impending strokes and often brightened up people who were suffering from cerebral vascular insufficiency.

Floyd died a few years ago, and I was very sorry to hear of it, but he must have been about 85, so he did pretty well.

FAITH

Many of my patients really seemed to believe that I could and would take care of anything that happened to them. On more than one occasion patients actually kissed my hand. That faith was not entirely justified, but I envied them because it must have been comforting to believe that . I had never had that kind of faith in anyone since I was about eight years old.

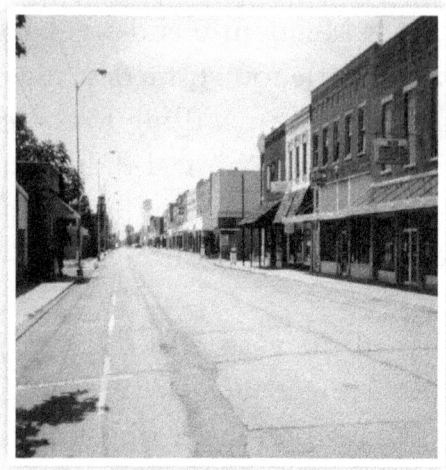

Fairbury Main Street

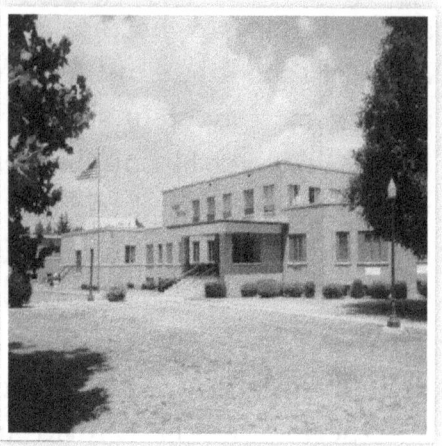

Fairbury Hospital

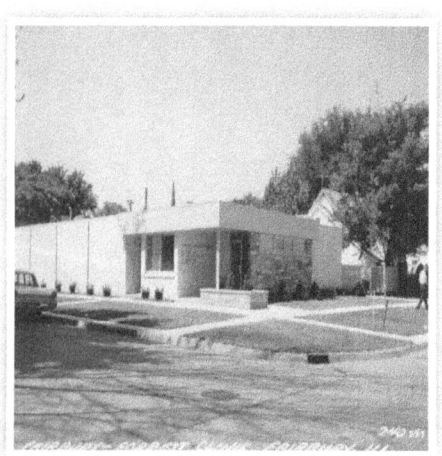

Fairbury Forrest Clinic

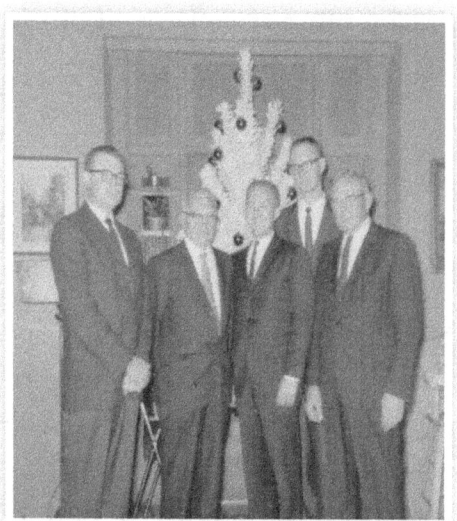

Drs. Ervin, Marshall,Hudgens,
Bort and Sauer

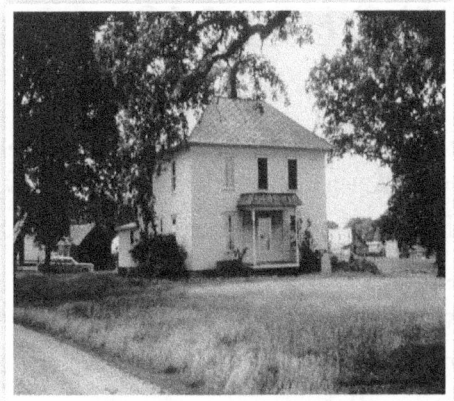

"Dream house" before

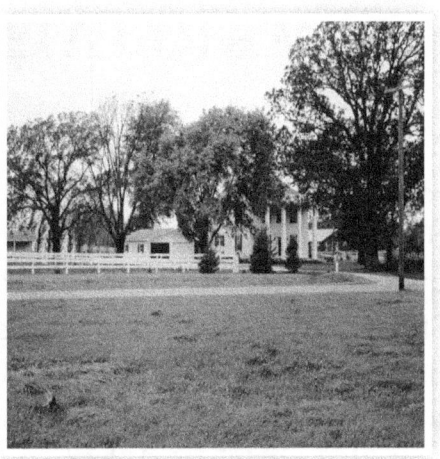

"Dream house" after

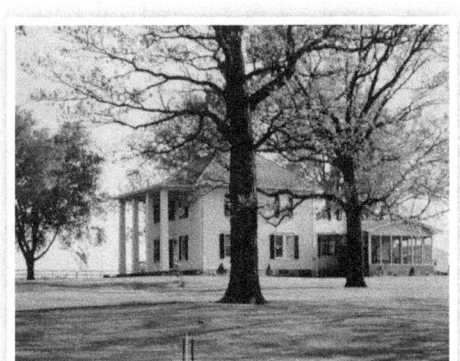

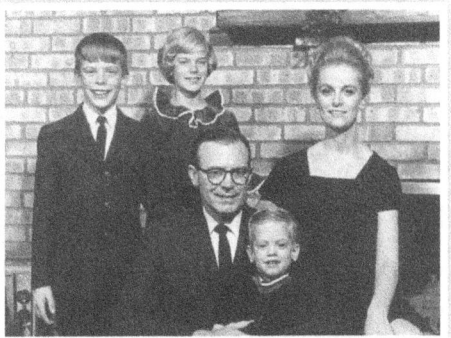

Dr. Ervin and family

MARITAL PROBLEMS

My wife was very attractive, but she was "high maintenance". She required a lot of attention and recognition and a lot of money, I thought, to indulge her whims. The first six or seven years of our marriage were actually pretty good, but then it started to deteriorate. She resented cooking and housework and became progressively more disagreeable. She was always coquettish and often outright flirtatious. She thought, with some justification, that she had some control over men, and she loved to exercise it. That annoyed me, but I didn't think it was a serious problem. In 1970 she enrolled in the junior college in Pontiac. When, in August of that year, I discovered that she was having a torrid sexual affair with a much younger male fellow student, I was completely devastated and heartbroken. My carefully built world came crashing down.

I told Glenn about the situation and told him that I had to leave town for a few days to figure out what to do. He was, as usual, agreeable. I considered divorce and actually had papers served on her, but I hated the thought of losing my children and half of everything I owned. My mother advised me to swallow my pride and try to keep my family together. When I returned home my wife denied everything and professed love for me, and, I'll admit, I was still attracted to her. She actually did have some control over men, including me.

I suggested that we move elsewhere and try to make a new start. Earlier that year I had bought a small ranch in Colorado, and we decided to move to Denver. Bob Bort had left earlier that summer for a residency in psychiatry, and Glenn and I had recruited another young partner who would join us when he got out of the army. I made arrangements to transfer my part of the practice to the new guy and traveled to Denver to buy a house and find a job. I also sold my "dream house" to a local lawyer.

In Denver we bought a nice house, and I took a job as one of twenty physicians in a city-owned clinic in a poor, mostly black neighborhood. For the next year I was very severely depressed. I had been cuckolded by my wife, and I had gone from being a highly respected, almost revered doctor, chief of staff at the hospital, president of the county medical society and delegate to the state medical society to being no one in particular. My income was cut by about two thirds. It wasn't possible to duplicate in Colorado the sort of practice I had built in Fairbury, and I was too depressed to even try.

A DIFFERENT KIND OF LIFE

After a few months I was asked to become the Medical Director of the clinic where I worked and to get involved in medical administration and public health. I was still very depressed, but I accepted for lack of anything better to do. In the years that followed I went back to school and got a masters degree in health administration and took increasingly more prestigious positions, but I would never again be the kind of doctor I had always wanted to be and had been for thirteen years.

On the other hand, it was very nice to work only forty hours each week instead of eighty, to be off every night and weekend and to go to bed knowing that I wouldn't have to get up until the next morning. Our marriage was fairly good for another year or so, but my wife's basic nature hadn't changed, and we were divorced a few years later. I felt, at that point, that I done all I could to keep our family together. My work in medical education and administration was mildly interesting, but the depression continued off and on for another six or eight years until I finally accepted the idea that there is more to life than work.

DON L. ERVIN, MD

THE NEIGHBORHOOD HEALTH PROGRAM

The clinic where I worked in Denver was part of the Neighborhood Health Program which had two major divisions, the East Side and the West Side. I worked on the East Side and soon became its Medical Director. We employed about twenty physicians, eight dentists and three hundred support staff. We had an annual budget of 4 .5 million dollars and were funded by the City of Denver and, mostly, by federal grants. This was during the time of Lyndon Johnson's War On Poverty. We had a large Health Center and four smaller Health Stations out in the community. My duties were mostly administrative. It was very inefficient. After about four years I realized that nothing I did could make it better or worse, and I became very bored. I also realized that the purpose of the program was less about providing health care and more about funneling federal (taxpayer) money into the community. When I was offered a position as Medical Director of the Rural Health Care Association I took it.

THE RURAL HEALTH CARE ASSOCIATION

This was a non-profit organization funded primarily by a grant from the Johnson Foundation. Its purpose was to develop and implement methods for improving health care in rural areas. Being at heart a country doctor, this sounded more interesting to me. As Medical Director my duties included designing facilities, purchasing equipment, training staff, recruiting physicians, monitoring quality of care and providing part time physician coverage when needed. This involved a lot of travel around Colorado in small planes and was pretty exciting. When our grant money ran out after about four years, I practiced alternate weeks in our facility in Yuma, Colorado for about a year. During that time I decided that I didn't want to be a country doctor anymore.

SAINT JOSEPH HOSPITAL

St. Joseph is a 560 bed Catholic hospital in Denver operated by the Sisters of Charity of Leavenworth. It is a very prestigious teaching hospital with residencies in Medicine, Surgery, OB and Family Practice. In 1979 I was asked to become Associate Director of the Family Practice Residency and accepted. It was a three year program with four residents in each year. After two years I became the Director and did that for four years before being promoted to Medical Vice President of the hospital. This was an entirely administrative position. I didn't like it much, but the fringe benefits were very good, and I decided to stick it out until I could retire with a pension, which I did. During my time at St. Joseph I was married again for about eight years, but that was not a good match, and the divorce was a merciful relief for both of us.

WALT

Walter Schreibman has been my solid, dependable friend for forty years. He was teaching psychology at a local community college in Lakewood, Colorado when we first met, and still is. About thirty years ago, when I was Director of the Family Practice Residency at St. Joseph Hospital, I asked him to become the Behavioral Science teacher for our residents, and he's still doing that too. In 1996 he and Sally Berger, one of our former residents, asked me to go with them on a medical mission to Zimbabwe, which I did. It was an incredibly rewarding and exciting experience and was the last time I was able to be a real doctor for awhile. He and Sally were married shortly after we returned, and she is now also a true and dependable friend. Walt helped me through some hard times with my divorces and has been very helpful with projects at the ranch, where we often go to fish and relax.

FAMILY

During the last thirty five years I have been able to spend a lot of time with my son Daniel and my daughter Ann. They have both grown into delightful, responsible adults with families of their own, and I have had many wonderful times with them and their children. I hope to have some more.

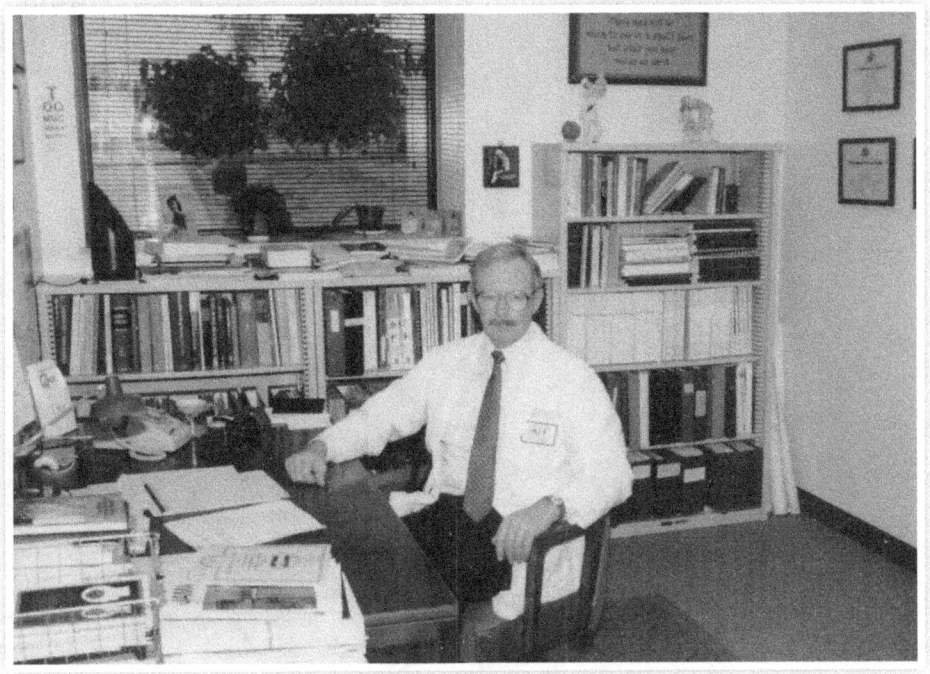

Family Practice Residency Director

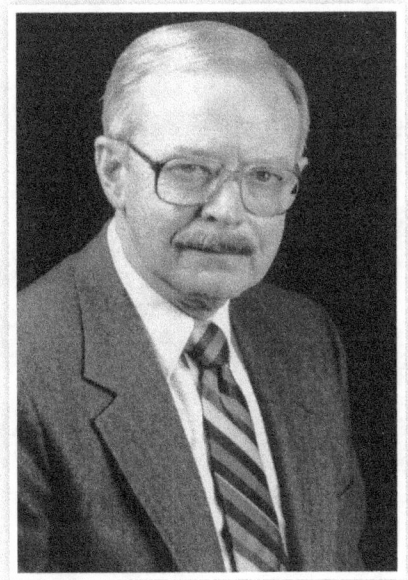

Vice President-St. Joseph Hospital

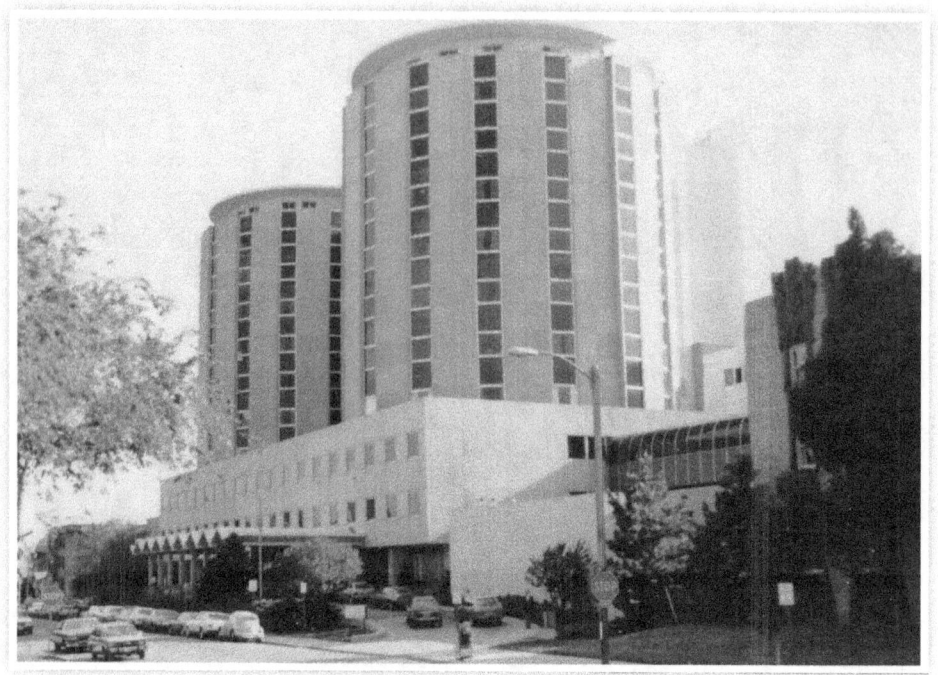

Saint Joseph Hospital, Denver, Colorado

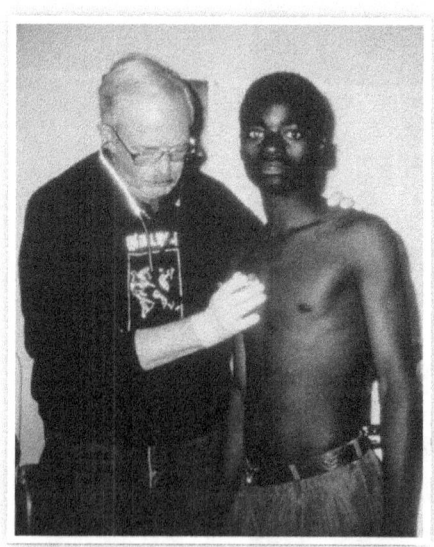

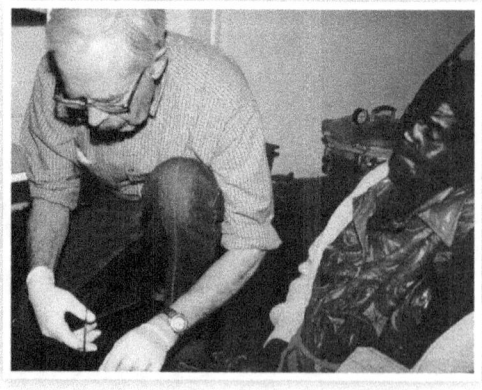

In Africa

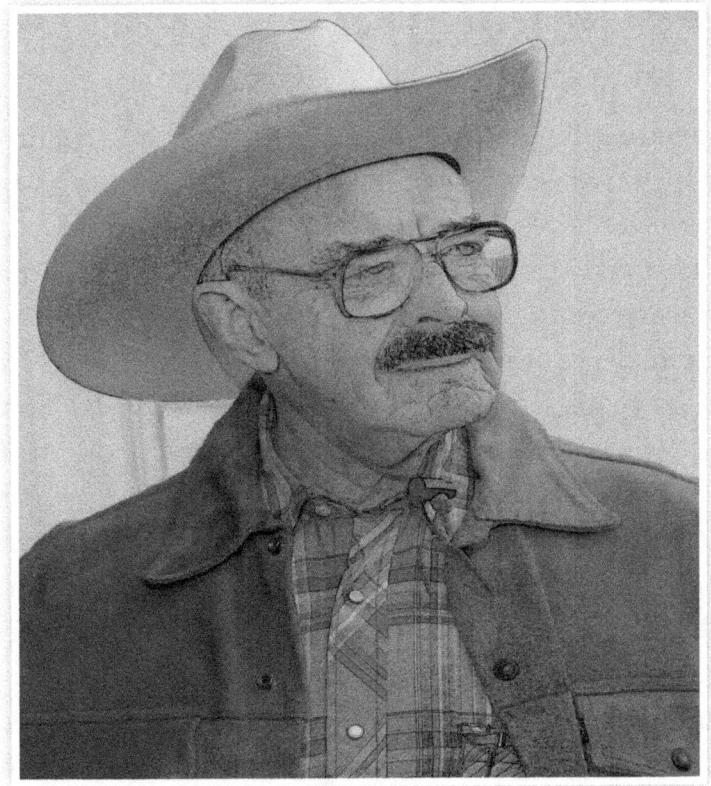

Rancher

DON L. ERVIN, MD

LOOKING BACK

Many remarkable changes in medical care have occurred over the past fifty five years, most of which have been improvements. Some, however, have not. Probably no one in America gets the kind of personal service we provided in Fairbury and never will again, and the cost of health care is clearly out of control. In spite of my extensive education and varied experience in the field, I'm not sure how this happened or what to do about it. Some of it, of course, is the result of inflation, and some is due to the cost of the complex equipment which we now can't do without. A lot, I believe, can be attributed to the system of "third party payers" which means health insurance and Medicare. This system has made it possible for patients to get treatments which they couldn't afford without it and has enriched some "health care providers". On the other hand, the doctors and patients care less about the cost when someone else is paying it, and it goes up...a lot. Another factor is liability insurance. I couldn't, today, do all of the OB and surgery I used to do in Fairbury, because the malpractice insurance would cost more than I made in a year. We can't reverse these things, and it will probably get worse before it gets better. However, as Winston Churchill said, America always does the right thing, after exhausting every other alternative.

I'm eternally grateful that I had the opportunity to be the kind of doctor I wanted to be for at least thirteen years.

www.ingramcontent.com/pod-product-compliance
Lightning Source LLC
Chambersburg PA
CBHW071619170526
45166CB00003B/1115